HAIR GROWTH ELIXIR: 100% Natural Hair Growth Solution!

Unlock the Beauty of Radiant Hair Growth: Discover the Secret to Thicker and Healthier Hair and Say Goodbye to Hair Loss Naturally Without Any Side Effects.

MRS. VERA JACOB

HAIR GROWTH ELIXIR: 100% Natural Hair Growth Solution! Copyright Notice. By Mrs. Vera Jacob

Contents

INTRODUCTION

In a world inundated with quick fixes and synthetic solutions, there remains an age-old treasure trove waiting to be rediscovered—the incredible power of natural remedies for hair growth. Welcome to a journey that celebrates the marvels of nature and the rejuvenating prowess it holds for our most prized crown—our hair.

The quest for luscious, vibrant hair isn't merely a pursuit of beauty; it's a testament to our inherent desire for vitality and well-being. "HAIR GROWTH ELIXIR: 100% Natural Hair Growth Solution!" is your gateway to understanding, embracing, and harnessing the potent gifts that nature offers to nurture and restore the glory of your locks.

Within these pages, you'll unearth a tapestry of holistic approaches, ancient wisdom, and modern scientific revelations woven together to create a comprehensive guide. From the gentle caress of herbal infusions to the nourishing touch of oils derived from nature's bounty, this book unveils the secrets that have sustained generations, offering remedies that work in harmony with your body's rhythms.

Whether you yearn for thicker, faster-growing strands, battle with hair loss, or simply seek to amplify the radiance of your mane, this book is your personalized roadmap. It's a testament to the versatility and effectiveness of natural remedies, tailored to fit diverse lifestyles and preferences.

Remember, nurturing your hair isn't just a routine—it's an intimate journey of self-care and discovery. As we embark together, we'll explore practices that transcend beyond external treatments, delving into the nuances of nutrition, mindfulness, and the holistic well-being of your hair and scalp. Let's embark on this empowering expedition together,

HAIR GROWTH ELIXIR: 100% Natural Hair Growth Solution! unlocking the abundance that nature offers and revitalizing our relationship with the hair that embodies our unique beauty.

CHAPTER ONE
Overview to a Healthier and Vibrant Hair

Welcome to the journey of embracing the natural essence of healthy, vibrant hair. In today's fast-paced world, where beauty trends come and go, the timeless allure of luxurious locks remains a symbol of vitality and confidence. This book, "HAIR GROWTH ELIXIR: 100% Natural Hair Growth Solution!," aims to be your trusted companion in navigating the realm of natural remedies and nurturing your hair from roots to tips.

Within these pages, you'll embark on a holistic exploration of botanical wonders, ancient remedies, and modern scientific insights, all tailored to enhance the natural growth and strength of your hair. As we delve into this realm, we'll unravel the mysteries of various herbs, oils, nutrients, and practices that have stood the test of time, empowering you

HAIR GROWTH ELIXIR: 100% Natural Hair Growth Solution!

to reclaim the health and radiance of your hair in harmony with nature.

Whether you're seeking solutions for thinning hair, aiming for faster growth, or simply striving to maintain the luster of your mane, this book is designed to be your go-to resource. It's crafted to provide practical, easy-to-implement strategies that harmonize with diverse lifestyles and preferences.

Remember, the path to healthier hair isn't just about external treatments; it's a holistic approach that encompasses nourishment, self-care, and understanding the individual needs of your hair and scalp. With this book, I invite you to embark on a journey of self-discovery, empowerment, and natural beauty, one that celebrates the innate magnificence of your hair.

HAIR GROWTH ELIXIR: 100% Natural Hair Growth Solution!
Let's embark together on this transformative voyage toward
radiant, naturally flourishing hair!

Understanding Hair Growth

Hair is not just dead cells; it is a testament to the intricacies of our body's functions and cycles. Understanding the fundamentals of hair growth is crucial to unlocking the secrets of nurturing healthy and flourishing locks.

The Hair Growth Cycle

Hair growth is a dynamic process governed by a cycle comprising three key phases: anagen, catagen, and telogen.

The **anagen phase** is the active growth phase, where hair cells divide rapidly, leading to new hair formation. This phase can last anywhere from two to seven years, determining the length of your hair.

Following anagen comes the **catagen phase**, a transitional period lasting about two weeks. During this phase, hair stops growing and detaches from the blood supply, signaling the end of active growth.

Lastly, the **telogen phase** is the resting phase that spans roughly three months. Hair follicles remain dormant before shedding and restarting the cycle anew.

Numerous internal and external factors influence this intricate cycle. Genetics play a pivotal role in determining hair growth patterns, influencing hair thickness, texture, and potential balding. Additionally, hormonal changes, stress levels, diet, and overall health significantly impact the hair growth process.

Understanding your unique hair type is a foundational step toward effective hair care. Hair textures vary—ranging from straight to curly to kinky—and each demands specific care routines. Likewise, individual scalp conditions and sensitivities require tailored attention.

To accurately cater to your hair's needs, assessing its porosity, moisture levels, and scalp health is imperative. This knowledge forms the bedrock upon which you'll craft a personalized regimen using natural treatments to optimize growth and vitality.

Comprehending the intricate dance of the hair growth cycle, recognizing influential factors, and deciphering your hair's unique traits are pivotal in crafting a holistic approach to nurturing your hair naturally.

This section sets the stage by providing essential knowledge about the hair growth cycle, the factors impacting it, and the importance of understanding one's unique hair type and needs for effective natural treatment strategies.

Factors Affecting Hair Growth

The quest for healthier, more vibrant hair isn't solely reliant on external treatments—it's a harmonious interplay between internal health, lifestyle choices, and environmental factors. Understanding the myriad influences on hair growth is pivotal in devising a holistic approach toward nurturing your locks naturally.

1. Genetics: The Blueprint of Your Hair

Your genetic makeup plays a significant role in determining hair characteristics. Family history often dictates hair texture, density, and potential hair loss patterns. While genetics set the foundation, they aren't the sole dictators of your hair's destiny. Natural treatments can complement and optimize the innate traits of your hair.

2. **Hormonal Balance: The Orchestra Conductor**

Hormones wield considerable influence over hair growth cycles. Fluctuations in hormonal levels, such as during puberty, pregnancy, or menopause, can impact hair growth. Conditions like polycystic ovary syndrome (PCOS) or thyroid disorders can also affect hair health by disrupting hormonal balance.

3. **Nutrit3ion and Diet: Feeding Your Follicles**

The adage "you are what you eat" resonates profoundly in the context of hair health. A diet rich in essential nutrients like protein, vitamins (particularly A, C, D, and E), minerals (like iron and zinc), and omega-3 fatty acids is vital for promoting healthy hair growth. Deficiencies can hinder hair follicle function, leading to issues like hair thinning or breakage.

4. Stress and Lifestyle: Mind-Body Connection

Stress isn't merely a mental state—it reflects in your hair health too. Elevated stress levels trigger hormonal imbalances that can lead to hair shedding or stunted growth. Additionally, lifestyle factors such as smoking, excessive alcohol consumption, and lack of sleep can adversely impact hair vitality.

5. Environmental Factors: External Challenges

Exposure to environmental pollutants, UV radiation, harsh chemicals in hair care products, and heat styling tools can damage the hair cuticle, leading to brittleness, dryness, and breakage. Protecting your hair from these external stressors is vital for maintaining its health and promoting growth.

Understanding these multifaceted factors enables you to identify potential challenges and tailor a natural treatment regimen that addresses these influences, fostering an environment conducive to optimal hair growth and vitality.

Identifying Your Hair Type And Needs

Understanding the unique characteristics and needs of your hair is a pivotal step in crafting an effective natural treatment regimen. Your hair type, texture, and individual scalp conditions determine the specific care it requires for optimal growth and vitality.

1. Hair Texture: The Foundation of Care

Hair textures vary widely, spanning from straight to wavy, curly, and curly. Identifying your hair's texture helps determine the products and routines best suited for it. Straight hair tends to be oilier at the scalp, while curly or curly hair may be drier due to the natural oils struggling to travel down the strands.

2. Porosity: Understanding Absorption

Low porosity hair repels moisture, making it challenging to hydrate, while high porosity hair readily absorbs moisture but struggles to retain it. Conducting a simple porosity test, like the water test or the slip and slide test, aids in understanding your hair's porosity level.

3. Scalp Health: The Foundation of Growth

A healthy scalp is the fertile ground from which healthy hair grows. Conditions like dandruff, scalp inflammation, or excessive oiliness can impede hair growth. Assessing your scalp's condition allows for targeted treatments to address specific issues and create an environment conducive to optimal growth.

4. Needs Assessment: Tailoring Your Routine

Once you've identified your hair type and scalp condition, you can curate a personalized regimen. For instance, dry or curly hair may benefit from deep conditioning treatments, while oily scalps might require more frequent cleansing with gentle, natural products.

5. Adapting to Change: Hair's Dynamic Nature

It's essential to note that hair needs can evolve over time due to factors like seasonal changes, hormonal shifts, or lifestyle alterations. Regularly reassessing your hair's needs allows for adjustments in your natural treatment routine to accommodate these fluctuations.

By recognizing and embracing the unique attributes of your hair, you pave the way for a tailored natural treatment approach that caters precisely to its requirements, nurturing it from root to tip for enhanced growth and vibrancy.

HAIR GROWTH ELIXIR: 100% Natural Hair Growth Solution!

This section aims to empower readers to understand their hair's unique traits and needs, facilitating the customization of a natural treatment regimen that optimally supports their hair growth journey.

CHAPTER TWO
Nourishing From Within

Achieving vibrant, healthy hair isn't solely about external treatments; it begins from within. Providing your body with the essential nutrients it needs sets the foundation for robust, flourishing hair growth.

A balanced diet rich in essential nutrients serves as the cornerstone for vibrant hair. Proteins, essential fatty acids, vitamins, and minerals play pivotal roles in supporting hair health. Incorporating lean proteins like fish, chicken, beans, and nuts ensures an adequate supply of amino acids necessary for hair structure and growth.

Supplements can complement your diet to address any nutritional gaps that might affect hair health. Biotin, known as vitamin B7, is particularly recognized for its role in promoting healthy hair growth. Additionally, vitamins A, C,

D, and E, along with minerals like iron and zinc, contribute significantly to hair vitality.

1. Hydration for Hair Health

Hydration is fundamental not just for your body but also for your hair. Drinking ample water keeps your scalp and hair follicles hydrated, promoting a healthy environment for hair growth. Dehydration can make your hair brittle and prone to breakage, emphasizing the importance of maintaining adequate hydration levels.

2. Balancing Act: Diet and Lifestyle

A balanced lifestyle and a nutritious diet go hand in hand. Stress management techniques, regular exercise, and adequate sleep positively impact overall health, consequently benefiting hair growth. Stress reduction is particularly crucial, as chronic stress can disrupt hormonal balance, leading to hair problems.

3. Mindful Eating for Hair Growth

Practicing mindful eating habits ensures that you're not just consuming nutrients but also absorbing them effectively. Slow down, savor your meals, and focus on nutrient-dense foods to maximize their benefits for your hair and overall well-being.

By nourishing your body from within with a wholesome diet, adequate hydration, and mindful lifestyle practices, you lay the groundwork for promoting robust hair growth and maintaining its vibrancy naturally. This segment emphasizes the significance of internal nourishment for healthy hair growth, covering aspects of nutrition, supplementation, hydration, and lifestyle habits to support readers in fostering a conducive environment for optimal hair health.

Supplements and Vitamins For Hair Growth

In the pursuit of healthy, luscious hair, supplements and vitamins can serve as valuable allies. While a balanced diet forms the foundation for optimal hair health, certain supplements and vitamins can supplement nutritional needs and promote robust hair growth.

1. Biotin (Vitamin B7):

Biotin is renowned for its role in enhancing hair growth and strength. This water-soluble vitamin aids in the production of keratin, a protein vital for healthy hair. Foods like eggs, nuts, and leafy greens are natural sources, but supplementing with biotin might further support hair health, especially for individuals with biotin deficiencies.

2. Vitamin A:

Vitamin A plays a crucial role in aiding the scalp's production of sebum, an oily substance that moisturizes the scalp and keeps hair healthy. It's pivotal for cell growth and differentiation, promoting a healthy scalp environment for optimal hair growth. Natural sources like sweet potatoes, carrots, and spinach offer vitamin A, but excessive intake can have adverse effects, so moderation is key.

3. Vitamin C:

This antioxidant vitamin contributes to collagen production, which is essential for maintaining hair strength and elasticity.

4. Vitamin D:

Research suggests a link between vitamin D deficiency and hair loss. Adequate levels of vitamin D support hair follicle growth cycles, making it an important vitamin for overall hair health. Exposure to sunlight is a natural way to increase vitamin D levels, alongside fortified foods and supplements.

5. Vitamin E:

Vitamin E is known for its antioxidant properties, helping to reduce oxidative stress in the scalp. It aids in improving blood circulation, promoting a healthy scalp environment conducive to hair growth. Nuts, seeds, and leafy greens are natural sources of vitamin E.

6. Iron and Zinc:

Iron is vital for carrying oxygen to hair follicles, while zinc supports hair tissue growth and repair. Red meat, beans, lentils, and seeds are good sources of iron and zinc.

Before starting any supplementation regimen, it's advisable to consult with a healthcare professional to assess individual needs and ensure the supplements are safe and suitable. While supplements can complement a healthy diet, they are not a substitute for a balanced nutrition plan.

Hydration and Its Impact On Hair

Hydration is not just essential for overall health—it's a cornerstone of vibrant, healthy hair. Adequate hydration plays a pivotal role in maintaining the moisture balance of your scalp and hair strands, directly influencing their health and growth.

1. Scalp Health: The Foundation

The scalp, like the skin elsewhere on your body, requires hydration to function optimally. A well-hydrated scalp fosters an environment conducive to healthy hair growth. Insufficient hydration can lead to dryness, flakiness, and irritation, potentially hindering the hair growth cycle.

2. Moisture Retention: For Stronger Strands

Hair strands, primarily composed of keratin, rely on moisture for strength and flexibility. Well-hydrated hair is less prone to breakage, splitting, and brittleness. Moisture retention within the hair shafts ensures they remain supple and less susceptible to damage from external stressors.

3. Preventing Dryness: A Key to Luster

Dry hair lacks the natural shine and luster associated with healthy hair. Adequate hydration helps seal the hair cuticle, preventing moisture loss and enhancing the reflective properties of the hair, resulting in a more vibrant appearance.

4. Balancing Act: External and Internal Hydration

Hydration for your hair involves both internal and external factors. Drinking sufficient water ensures that your body can hydrate your scalp and hair from within. Additionally, using hydrating, natural hair care products, and incorporating conditioning treatments aids in external hydration, maintaining moisture levels in your hair.

5. Tips for Hydration:

i. **Drink Water:** Aim to maintain optimal hydration levels by drinking enough water daily.

ii. **Use Hydrating Products:** Choose natural, moisturizing shampoos and conditioners that nourish your hair without stripping away natural oils.

iii. **Deep Conditioning:** Incorporate regular deep conditioning treatments or masks containing hydrating ingredients like aloe vera, coconut oil, or honey to infuse moisture into your hair.

6. Conclusion

Hydration is a fundamental aspect of healthy hair growth. By ensuring your scalp and hair strands are adequately hydrated from both internal and external sources, you

HAIR GROWTH ELIXIR: 100% Natural Hair Growth Solution! provide the ideal conditions for strong, resilient, and lustrous hair.

CHAPTER THREE
Herbal Remedies

Nature's bounty offers a wealth of herbal remedies rich in nutrients, antioxidants, and natural compounds that have been revered for centuries for their ability to nourish, strengthen, and stimulate hair growth. Incorporating these herbal remedies into your hair care routine can promote healthier, more resilient hair.

Herbs for Strengthening and Growth
1. Amla (Indian Gooseberry):

Rich in vitamin C and antioxidants, amla promotes hair growth, strengthens hair follicles, and helps maintain scalp health. Amla oil or powder can be applied to the scalp or consumed orally to benefit from its properties.

2. Aloe Vera:

Renowned for its soothing and moisturizing properties, aloe vera contains enzymes that promote hair growth, reduce scalp inflammation, and maintain the scalp's pH balance. Applying aloe vera gel directly to the scalp can nourish hair follicles and encourage growth.

3. Rosemary:

Rosemary aid in stimulating the circulation in the scalp, thereby promoting hair growth and preventing any form of hair loss. Its antifungal properties also contribute to a healthier scalp. Infusing rosemary leaves in oil or using rosemary essential oil in a scalp massage can be beneficial.

4. Fenugreek (Methi):

Fenugreek seeds are rich in proteins and nicotinic acid, which strengthen hair and promote growth. Soaking fenugreek seeds overnight and blending them into a paste

HAIR GROWTH ELIXIR: 100% Natural Hair Growth Solution!

for a scalp treatment can improve hair texture and encourage growth.

5. Horsetail (Equisetum arvense):

Horsetail contains silica, a mineral that strengthens hair strands and stimulates growth. Using horsetail extract or tea as a rinse can contribute to healthier, more resilient hair.

6. Hibiscus:

Hibiscus flowers are rich in vitamins and amino acids that nourish hair, prevent premature graying, and strengthen hair follicles. Creating a hair mask or oil infusion using hibiscus flowers can promote hair growth and shine.

7. Neem:

Neem's antifungal and antibacterial properties help maintain a healthy scalp by combating dandruff and other scalp conditions that might hinder hair growth. Using neem oil or neem-infused products can promote a healthier scalp environment.

8. Coconut Oil:

While not an herb, coconut oil is a potent natural remedy for hair growth. Its fatty acids penetrate the hair shaft, preventing protein loss and keeping hair hydrated. Massaging warm coconut oil into the scalp can promote growth and overall hair health.

Incorporating these herbal remedies into your hair care routine allows you to harness the nourishing, strengthening, and growth-stimulating properties of nature, promoting healthy and resilient hair growth.

Essential Oils for Hair Health

Essential oils, derived from plants and renowned for their therapeutic properties, have long been treasured for their ability to nourish the scalp, promote hair growth, and enhance overall hair health. When used properly, these potent oils can be an excellent addition to your hair care routine.

1. Lavender Oil:

Lavender oil possesses antimicrobial properties that can improve scalp health by reducing dandruff and itching. Its calming scent also aids in stress reduction, which can indirectly benefit hair growth.

2. Peppermint Oil:

Peppermint oil is known for its cooling sensation and ability to stimulate blood circulation in the scalp. This enhanced circulation may promote hair growth by

HAIR GROWTH ELIXIR: 100% Natural Hair Growth Solution!

encouraging hair follicles to receive more nutrients and

oxygen.

3. Rosemary Oil:

Rosemary oil is celebrated for its ability to strengthen hair

follicles, improve circulation, and combat hair loss. It's a

versatile oil that can be used in scalp massages or added to

hair care products.

4. Cedarwood Oil:

Cedarwood oil aids in balancing oil production in the

scalp, making it beneficial for both dry and oily scalps. By

promoting a healthier scalp environment, it supports

optimal conditions for hair growth.

5. Tea Tree Oil:

Tea tree oil's antifungal and antibacterial properties make

it effective in treating various scalp conditions like

HAIR GROWTH ELIXIR: 100% Natural Hair Growth Solution!

dandruff and seborrheic dermatitis. Its cleansing properties

help maintain a healthy scalp.

6. Thyme Oil:

Thyme oil contains thymol, which has been linked to

improved hair growth by stimulating blood flow to the

scalp. It's often used in scalp treatments to enhance hair

thickness and growth.

7. Clary Sage Oil:

Clary sage oil regulates oil production in the scalp, making

it beneficial for both dry and oily hair types. It also

contains natural phytoestrogens that may support hair

growth.

8. Ylang-Ylang Oil:

HAIR GROWTH ELIXIR: 100% Natural Hair Growth Solution! Ylang-ylang oil's balancing properties can help soothe a dry or itchy scalp, contributing to a healthier scalp environment for improved hair growth.

When using essential oils, it's crucial to dilute them with carrier oils like coconut, jojoba, or almond oil to prevent skin irritation. Conduct a patch test and use these oils sparingly, as their potency requires careful application.

Do-It-Yourself (Diy) Herbal Treatments

Harnessing the power of herbs in DIY treatments offers a personalized, natural approach to nurturing hair growth. These simple, homemade remedies using herbs can provide nourishment, strengthen hair follicles, and stimulate healthy hair growth.

1. Herbal Infused Oils:

HAIR GROWTH ELIXIR: 100% Natural Hair Growth Solution!

Create herbal-infused oils by steeping herbs like rosemary, lavender, or thyme in carrier oils such as coconut or jojoba oil. Allow the herbs to infuse for a few weeks, strain, and use the oil for scalp massages to stimulate circulation and promote hair growth.

2. Herbal Hair Rinse:

Prepare an herbal hair rinse by steeping herbs like chamomile, nettle, or horsetail in hot water. This herbal infusion can nourish the scalp and strengthen hair strands.

3. Herbal Hair Masks:

Blend herbs like amla, hibiscus, fenugreek, or aloe vera into a paste using water or natural yoghurt. Apply this herbal mask to your scalp and hair, leaving it on for about 30 minutes before washing it off. These masks can nourish the scalp and promote hair growth.

4. Herbal Hair Sprays:

Create herbal hair sprays by infusing herbs like rosemary or lavender in water and using the strained liquid as a refreshing and nourishing spray for your scalp and hair.

5. Herbal Tea Rinses:

Brew herbal teas using herbs such as green tea, sage, or peppermint. After cooling, use the herbal tea as a rinse after shampooing to revitalize the scalp and promote healthier hair.

6. Herbal Scalp Massage Oils:

Combine essential oils with infused herbal oils for scalp massages. Lavender, rosemary, and peppermint essential oils are excellent choices for stimulating the scalp and promoting hair growth.

7. Herbal Vinegar Rinse:

HAIR GROWTH ELIXIR: 100% Natural Hair Growth Solution! Infuse herbs like rosemary, sage, or thyme in apple cider vinegar for several days. Dilute this herbal-infused vinegar with water and use it as a final hair rinse to restore pH balance and promote hair health.

When creating DIY herbal treatments, ensure to use fresh or dried herbs from reputable sources. Perform patch tests before using any new herbal treatment to avoid adverse reactions. Consistency and regular use of these herbal remedies can contribute to healthier, more vibrant hair.

CHAPTER FOUR
Holistic Practices

Achieving and maintaining healthy hair isn't solely about external treatments—it's a holistic journey that encompasses nourishment, self-care, and a harmonious balance of mind, body, and spirit. Integrating holistic practices into your routine supports overall well-being, creating an optimal environment for vibrant hair growth.

Regular scalp massages stimulate blood flow to the hair follicles, encouraging nutrient delivery and promoting hair growth. Incorporate gentle massage techniques using fingertips or a scalp massage tool to invigorate the scalp and relax the mind.

Chronic stress can disrupt hormonal balance, leading to hair loss or stunted growth. Practicing stress-reducing techniques like meditation, yoga, or deep breathing exercises can positively impact hair health by promoting relaxation and hormonal balance.

A well-rounded diet rich in nutrients—protein, vitamins, minerals, and healthy fats—is essential for healthy hair growth. Emphasize whole foods, lean proteins, leafy greens, and omega-3 fatty acids to nourish hair from within.

Limit the use of heat styling tools and chemical-laden hair products that can damage hair strands and dry out the scalp. Opt for natural hair care products free from harsh chemicals, and embrace protective hairstyles that minimize manipulation and breakage.

Regular physical activity improves blood circulation, including to the scalp, promoting healthier hair growth. Additionally, maintaining good sleep hygiene and staying hydrated are vital habits that positively impact overall health, reflecting in the quality of your hair.

Practicing mindfulness and self-care routines fosters a positive mindset, reducing stress and promoting overall well-being. Incorporate activities like journaling, hobbies, or simply dedicating time for relaxation to support mental and emotional health, indirectly benefiting hair health.

Environmental Considerations

Protect your hair from environmental stressors like pollution, UV rays, and harsh weather conditions. Wearing hats or scarves, using natural sun protection for hair, and rinsing hair after exposure to pool chlorine or salty sea water can help maintain hair health.

By embracing holistic practices that encompass nutrition, stress management, mindful self-care, and protective measures, you create a holistic environment that supports not only vibrant hair growth but also overall well-being.

Scalp Care and Massage Techniques

The scalp is the foundation for healthy hair growth, and proper care coupled with regular massages can significantly impact the vitality and strength of your hair follicles. Implementing scalp care and massage techniques into your routine can stimulate blood flow, nourish the scalp, and promote optimal conditions for hair growth.

1. Scalp Cleansing:

Use a gentle, natural shampoo to cleanse the scalp, removing excess oil, debris, and product buildup. Avoid harsh shampoos that strip the scalp of its natural oils, leading to dryness.

2. Gentle Brushing:

Using a soft-bristled brush, gently massage the scalp in circular motions. This stimulates blood flow and loosens dead skin cells, promoting a healthier scalp environment.

3. Proper Drying:

Avoid vigorous towel-drying that can cause friction and damage to wet hair. Instead, gently pat hair dry or opt for a microfiber towel to minimize friction and reduce breakage.

4. Scalp Massage Techniques:

i. **Fingertip Massage:** Use the pads of your fingers, not nails, to gently massage the scalp in circular motions. Start from the front hairline and work your way to the back, covering the entire scalp.

ii. **Kneading Massage:** With the pads of your fingers, apply gentle pressure and knead the scalp in small circular motions. This helps release tension and improves blood circulation to the hair follicles.

iii. **Essential Oil Massage:** Combine a few drops of essential oils (like lavender, rosemary, or peppermint) with a carrier oil (such as coconut or jojoba oil). Massage this mixture into the scalp for added nourishment and stimulation.

5. Frequency and Duration:

Ensure that scalp massages is incorporated into your daily activities, few times per week. Aim for at least 5-10 minutes per session to reap the benefits of improved circulation and relaxation.

6. Benefits of Scalp Massage:

i. Stimulates blood circulation, delivering nutrients and oxygen to hair follicles.

ii. Promotes relaxation and reduces stress, which can indirectly benefit hair health.

iii. Helps in the distribution of natural oils, keeping the scalp and hair moisturized.

7. Consistency and Patience:

Consistency is key in reaping the benefits of scalp massages. While results may not be immediate, regular massages can gradually improve scalp health and contribute to healthier hair over time.

Incorporating scalp care and massage into your routine not only enhances the health of your scalp but also promotes stronger, more resilient hair growth. It's a simple yet effective way to nurture your hair from its roots.

Stress Management for Healthy Hair

Stress isn't just an emotional state, it can manifest physically, affecting various bodily functions, including hair growth. Managing stress levels is crucial for maintaining healthy hair, as chronic stress can disrupt the hair growth cycle and lead to issues like hair loss or thinning.

1. Understanding the stress-hair relationship:

Stress triggers hormonal imbalances that affect the hair growth cycle. Excessive stress can push more hair follicles into the resting phase (telogen), leading to increased shedding or stunted growth.

2. Stress-Reducing Techniques:

i. **Mindfulness and Meditation:** Practicing mindfulness, meditation, or deep breathing exercises can help reduce stress levels. Taking a few minutes daily to relax and clear your mind can have positive effects on overall well-being, including hair health.

ii. **Regular Exercise:** Engaging in physical activity not only improves circulation, benefiting the scalp, but also releases endorphins that combat stress hormones. Find activities you enjoy to make exercise a stress-relieving habit.

iii. **Yoga or Tai Chi:** These practices combine movement with mindfulness, promoting relaxation and reducing stress. Certain poses or movements specifically target stress reduction, benefiting both mind and body.

3. Healthy Lifestyle Choices:

i. **Balanced Diet:** Consuming nutrient-rich foods supports overall health and can help combat the effects of stress on the body, indirectly benefiting hair health.

ii. **Adequate Sleep:** Quality sleep is crucial for stress management and overall health. Lack of sleep can exacerbate stress levels, impacting hair growth and quality.

4. Stress Reduction Techniques in Daily Life:

i. **Setting Boundaries:** Establishing boundaries and managing workload or commitments can reduce stress levels. Learning to say 'no' when necessary helps prevent overwhelming situations.

ii. **Time for Relaxation:** Dedicate time each day for activities that bring joy and relaxation, whether it's reading, hobbies, or spending time outdoors.

iii. **Seeking Support:** Talking to friends, family, or seeking professional help if stress becomes overwhelming can alleviate its impact on your life and consequently on hair health.

Managing stress isn't just beneficial for mental and emotional well-being—it's crucial for maintaining healthy hair growth. By adopting stress-reducing practices and making lifestyle adjustments, you create an environment conducive to optimal hair health.

Natural Styling and Hair Care Routine

Opting for natural styling and adopting a hair care routine that nurtures your hair without harsh chemicals or excessive heat can significantly contribute to healthier, more resilient hair growth.

1. **Gentle Cleansing with Natural Products:**

Choose gentle, natural shampoos and conditioners that cleanse without stripping away the scalp's natural oils. Look for sulfate-free and paraben-free products that nourish the hair and scalp without causing dryness or irritation.

2. **Proper Conditioning and Moisture Retention:**

Regular conditioning is essential for maintaining moisture in the hair. Consider deep conditioning treatments using natural ingredients like aloe vera, coconut oil, or shea butter to nourish and strengthen the hair shafts.

3. Minimize Heat Styling:

Limit the use of heat styling tools like straighteners or curling irons, as excessive heat can damage hair cuticles, leading to breakage and dryness. Opt for heatless styling methods like air-drying or braiding to achieve desired looks without heat damage.

4. Protective Hairstyles:

Embrace protective hairstyles that minimize manipulation and stress on hair strands. Braids, twists, buns, or gentle ponytails protect the ends and reduce breakage caused by friction with clothing or accessories.

5. Scalp Care:

Nourishing the scalp is crucial for healthy hair growth. Regularly massage the scalp to stimulate blood flow and distribute natural oils. Consider using natural oils like coconut, jojoba, or argan oil as part of a scalp massage routine.

6. Avoid Harsh Chemicals:

Steer clear of harsh chemical treatments like relaxers, bleaches, or harsh dyes that can weaken the hair shaft and cause damage. Opt for natural hair color options or henna-based dyes if coloring is desired.

7. Trim Regularly:

Trimming your hair on a regular basis has the potency to eliminate split ends and prevent additional damage.

HAIR GROWTH ELIXIR: 100% Natural Hair Growth Solution!

Trimming every few months can maintain healthy hair ends and promote overall hair health.

8. Protect Hair from Environmental Stressors:

Shield your hair from environmental stressors like sun exposure, wind, and pollution. Wearing hats or scarves can protect hair from UV rays and prevent damage.

9. Routine Adjustment with Seasons:

Regulate hair care pattern according to weather changes. For instance, during colder months, extra moisture may be needed to combat dryness.

10.Holistic Approach:

Remember, healthy hair starts from within. Maintain a balanced diet, stay hydrated, manage stress levels, and get adequate sleep—these factors contribute significantly to hair health.

HAIR GROWTH ELIXIR: 100% Natural Hair Growth Solution!

Adopting a natural hair care routine that focuses on gentle treatments, minimal manipulation, and holistic practices sets the stage for healthy, vibrant hair growth. Consistency and patience with these methods are key to achieving long-term hair health.

CHAPTER FIVE
Targeted Solutions

Tailoring specific treatments and targeted solutions to address individual hair concerns can significantly enhance the growth and overall health of your hair. These focused approaches cater to various issues that might hinder optimal hair growth.

1. **Scalp Treatments:**

    i. **Exfoliation:** Use gentle exfoliating treatments to remove dead skin cells and product buildup from the scalp, promoting a healthier environment for hair growth.

    ii. **Scalp Serums or Tonics:** Choose natural scalp serums or tonics enriched with ingredients like peptides, vitamins, or botanical extracts that nourish the scalp and stimulate hair follicles.

2. Nutrient-Rich Hair Masks:

Create nutrient-rich hair masks using ingredients such as eggs, avocado, honey, or yogurt. These masks provide essential vitamins and proteins that strengthen hair and encourage growth.

3. Ayurvedic Treatments:

Explore Ayurvedic treatments such as scalp massages with herbal oils like Brahmi or Bhringraj oil. These herbal remedies have been used for centuries to nourish the scalp and promote hair growth.

4. Micro needling or Derma Rolling:

Micro needling or derma rolling involves using a roller with tiny needles to create micro-injuries on the scalp,

HAIR GROWTH ELIXIR: 100% Natural Hair Growth Solution!

stimulating blood flow and encouraging the production of

collagen and hair growth factors.

5. **Herbal Supplements or Tea Rinses:**

Incorporate herbal supplements or herbal tea rinses

containing herbs like saw palmetto, nettle, or horsetail that

are known for their potential to support healthy hair growth.

6. **Professional Treatments:**

Consider professional treatments like laser therapy or

platelet-rich plasma (PRP) therapy administered by

qualified practitioners, which have shown promise in

stimulating hair follicles and promoting growth.

7. **Lifestyle Adjustments:**

Evaluate and adjust lifestyle factors that could impact hair

growth. This includes ensuring adequate hydration,

managing stress levels, and maintaining a balanced diet rich in hair-nourishing nutrients.

8. Regular Assessment and Adaptation:

Regularly assess the effectiveness of targeted treatments and adjust your regimen as needed. Hair needs can change due to factors like seasonal changes or lifestyle adjustments.

9. Consultation with Professionals:

Consult with a dermatologist or trichologist to identify underlying issues that may be hindering hair growth and to receive personalized recommendations for treatment.

By incorporating targeted solutions and treatments tailored to address specific concerns, you create a more focused approach to promoting healthy hair growth. Consistency and patience are key to observing the results of these targeted interventions.

Thinning Hair: Remedies and Regimens

Dealing with thinning hair requires a specialized approach that focuses on nourishing the scalp, fortifying hair follicles, and promoting thicker, healthier hair growth. Implementing targeted remedies and regimens can significantly aid in addressing thinning hair concerns.

1. **Scalp Nourishment:**

i. **Essential Oils:** Incorporate essential oils such as rosemary, cedarwood, or peppermint into scalp massages to stimulate circulation and revitalize hair follicles.

ii. **Scalp Serums:** Opt for natural scalp serums containing ingredients like castor oil, argan oil, or plant-based extracts that nourish the scalp and promote thicker hair.

1. **Nutrient-Rich Treatments:**

i. **Protein Treatments:** Use protein-rich hair masks or treatments containing ingredients like eggs, yogurt, or fenugreek to strengthen hair strands and add volume.

ii. **Vitamin Supplements:** Consider supplements containing biotin, vitamins A, C, D, and E, and minerals like iron and zinc to support hair health and combat thinning.

2. **Herbal Remedies:**

i. **Amla (Indian Gooseberry):** Amla oil or powder contains antioxidants and vitamin C, which can strengthen hair and contribute to thicker, healthier strands.

ii. **Fenugreek Seed Paste:** Create a paste using fenugreek seeds and water or coconut milk and apply it to the scalp to boost hair volume and thickness.

3. **Lifestyle Adjustments:**

    i.   **Dietary Changes:** Focus on a balanced diet rich in proteins, healthy fats, and vitamins to nourish hair from within.

    ii. **Stress Management:** Practice stress-reducing techniques such as meditation or yoga to prevent stress-induced hair thinning.

4. **Scalp Stimulation Techniques:**

    i.   **Derma Rolling:** Consider using a derma roller to stimulate blood flow to the scalp, encouraging hair growth and enhancing absorption of topical treatments.

ii. **Low-Level Laser Therapy (LLLT):** Explore LLLT devices that have shown promise in improving hair density and thickness.

5. **Gentle Hair Care Practices:**

i. **Avoid Overstyling:** Minimize the use of heat styling tools and harsh chemicals that can further weaken fragile hair.

ii. **Regular Trimming:** Schedule regular trims to eliminate split ends and prevent breakage, maintaining the appearance of thicker hair.

6. **Professional Guidance:**

Consult with a dermatologist or trichologist to identify the underlying cause of thinning hair and receive personalized recommendations for treatment.

Consistency and dedication to a tailored regimen aimed at nourishing the scalp, strengthening hair, and addressing

HAIR GROWTH ELIXIR: 100% Natural Hair Growth Solution!

underlying causes of thinning can significantly improve hair

density and promote healthier, fuller-looking hair.

Combatting Hair Loss Naturally

Hair loss can be distressing, but several natural approaches

can help address this concern by nurturing the scalp,

strengthening hair follicles, and promoting healthy hair

growth without resorting to harsh chemicals or invasive

procedures.

1. **Scalp Nourishment:**

    i. **Scalp Massages:** Regularly massage the

       scalp using gentle pressure to stimulate

       blood circulation and encourage nutrient

       delivery to the hair follicles.

    ii. **Essential Oils:** Utilize essential oils like

       lavender, rosemary, or cedarwood in scalp

massages or as part of a natural treatment regimen to promote hair growth.

2. **Herbal Remedies:**

   i.   **Aloe Vera:** Apply aloe vera gel directly to the scalp to soothe inflammation, balance pH levels, and promote hair growth.

   ii. **Onion Juice:** Consider onion juice as a topical treatment; its sulfur content may aid in improving hair growth.

3. **Dietary Adjustments:**

   i.   **Protein-Rich Diet:** Ensure your diet includes sufficient proteins from sources like eggs, lean meats, legumes, and nuts, which are essential for hair growth.

   ii. **Omega-3 Fatty Acids:** Consume foods rich in omega-3s, such as salmon, flaxseeds, or walnuts, to support scalp health and reduce inflammation.

4. **Herbal Supplements:**

    i. **Biotin:** Consider taking biotin supplements, known to promote hair growth and improve hair structure.

    ii. **Saw Palmetto:** This herbal supplement may help block the formation of dihydrotestosterone (DHT), a hormone linked to hair loss in some individuals.

5. **Stress Reduction:**

    i. **Stress Management Techniques:** Engage in stress-relieving activities like meditation, yoga, or deep breathing exercises to reduce stress-induced hair loss.

    ii.   **Adequate Sleep:** Prioritize quality sleep to support overall health and mitigate the effects of stress on hair.

6. Lifestyle Modifications:

i.   **Gentle Hair Care:** Avoid harsh treatments, excessive heat styling, and tight hairstyles that can weaken hair and contribute to breakage.

ii.   **Regular Exercise:** Maintain a regular exercise routine to improve blood circulation, including to the scalp, supporting hair growth.

7. Consistency and Patience:

Consistency is key when adopting natural remedies for hair loss. Results may take time, so patience and persistence with the chosen regimen are essential.

8. Professional Consultation:

If hair loss persists or worsens, seek advice from a dermatologist or trichologist to identify any underlying conditions and receive tailored guidance.

By embracing natural remedies and holistic approaches, you can create a nurturing environment for your hair, promoting healthier growth and potentially combating hair loss without resorting to harsh interventions.

Promoting Faster Hair Growth

While hair growth rate is largely determined by genetics, there are natural methods and practices that can encourage and support faster hair growth by optimizing scalp health and nourishing hair follicles.

1. **Scalp Stimulation:**

i. **Scalp Massages:** Regularly massage the scalp to increase blood circulation, delivering essential nutrients to the hair follicles and promoting faster growth.

ii. **Exfoliation:** Gentle exfoliation of the scalp removes dead skin cells and buildup, allowing for unhindered hair growth.

2. **Nutrient-Rich Diet:**

iii. **Protein Intake:** Ensure adequate consumption of protein-rich foods like eggs, fish, beans, and nuts, as proteins are the building blocks of hair.

iv. **Vitamins and Minerals:** Incorporate foods rich in vitamins A, C, E, and biotin, as well as minerals like iron and zinc, which support hair growth and scalp health.

3. **Herbal Treatments:**

i. **Amla (Indian Gooseberry):** Consider using amla oil or consuming amla supplements, known for their hair-strengthening and growth-promoting properties.

ii. **Rosemary Oil:** Use rosemary oil in scalp massages to stimulate circulation and encourage faster hair growth.

4. **Hydration and Moisture:**

i. **Water Intake:** Stay adequately hydrated to support overall health, including hair health.

ii. **Natural Moisturizers:** Use natural oils like coconut, argan, or jojoba oil to moisturize the hair and scalp, preventing dryness and promoting growth.

5. **Scalp Masks and Treatments:**

i. **Hair Masks:** Apply homemade masks containing ingredients like yogurt, honey, or aloe vera, which nourish the scalp and encourage hair growth.

ii. **Herbal Rinses:** Rinse hair with herbal infusions like green tea or sage to stimulate follicles and enhance growth.

6. **Stress Management:**

i. **Relaxation Techniques:** Practice stress-relieving activities like yoga, meditation, or mindfulness to minimize stress-induced hair loss and encourage growth.

ii. **Adequate Sleep:** Ensure sufficient sleep to support the body's natural repair processes, including those involved in hair growth.

7. **Avoidance of Hair Stressors:**

i. **Heat and Chemicals:** Minimize the use of heat styling tools and harsh chemical treatments that can damage hair and slow growth.

ii. **Protective Styles:** Opt for protective hairstyles that prevent excessive pulling or tension on the hair, minimizing breakage and aiding growth.

8. **Regular Trimming:**

Trim hair regularly to remove split ends and prevent further damage, allowing for healthier hair growth from the roots.

By integrating these natural practices into a consistent routine and lifestyle, it's possible to create an environment conducive to faster hair growth while nurturing the scalp and supporting overall hair health.

CHAPTER SIX
Lifestyle and Maintenance

A holistic approach to hair care involves embracing a healthy lifestyle while maintaining consistent practices that support optimal hair growth. Incorporating specific habits and routines into your daily life can significantly contribute to healthier, stronger, and more vibrant hair.

1. Balanced Diet and Hydration:

i. **Nutrient-Rich Foods:** Consume a well-balanced diet consisting of proteins, vitamins (especially A, C, and E), minerals (like iron and zinc), and omega-3 fatty acids to nourish hair from within.

ii. **Hydration:** Stay adequately hydrated by drinking enough water daily to maintain scalp and hair health.

2. Stress Management:

i. **Stress-Reducing Activities:** Engage in activities like yoga, meditation, or deep breathing exercises to manage stress levels, which can impact hair health.

ii. **Adequate Rest:** Prioritize quality sleep to support overall health and aid in the body's natural hair growth cycle.

3. Gentle Hair Care Practices:

i. **Regular Washing:** Keep hair and scalp clean, but avoid overwashing, which can strip natural oils. Use mild, natural shampoos and conditioners suitable for your hair type.

ii. **Avoid Heat Damage:** Minimize the use of heat styling tools and opt for air-drying or heatless styling methods to prevent damage.

4. Scalp Care:

i. **Scalp Massages:** Incorporate regular scalp massages to stimulate blood flow and promote a healthy environment for hair growth.

ii. **Natural Oils:** Use natural oils like coconut, olive, or argan oil to moisturize and nourish the scalp and hair strands.

5. Protective Styling:

i. **Gentle Hairstyles:** Avoid tight hairstyles that pull on the hair, causing breakage. Opt for protective styles like braids or buns that minimize tension.

ii. **Headwear Protection:** Wear hats or scarves to shield hair from environmental stressors like sun exposure or harsh weather conditions.

6. Regular Trims:

Schedule regular trims every few months to remove split ends and prevent further damage, promoting healthier-looking hair.

7. Lifestyle Assessments:

Regularly evaluate lifestyle factors that could impact hair health, such as diet changes, stress levels, or environmental influences, and make necessary adjustments.

8. Professional Care:

Seek advice from a dermatologist or trichologist for personalized guidance and treatment plans if experiencing persistent issues with hair health.

Consistency and patience with these lifestyle and maintenance practices are crucial. By incorporating these habits into your daily routine, you create a conducive environment for promoting healthy hair growth and maintaining strong, resilient strands.

Healthy Habits for Beautiful Hair

Maintaining beautiful, lustrous hair involves adopting healthy habits that nurture both the scalp and hair strands. Incorporating these practices into your routine promotes stronger, shinier, and more vibrant hair.

1. Balanced Nutrition:

A nutrient-rich diet plays a fundamental role in promoting healthy hair. Ensure your meals include:

i. **Proteins**
ii. **Vitamins:** Particularly A, C, and E from fruits, vegetables, and nuts.
iii. **Minerals:** Including iron, zinc, and selenium from sources like spinach, nuts, and seeds.

iv. **Omega-3 Fatty Acids:** is one of the potent nutrients that walnuts, fish, and flaxseeds has.

2. Hydration:

Drink adequate water daily to keep your scalp and hair hydrated, preventing dryness and brittleness.

3. Gentle Hair Care:

i. **Regular Washing:** Use a gentle, sulfate-free shampoo suitable for your hair type and avoid washing excessively to maintain natural oils.

ii. **Conditioning:** Apply conditioner to the lengths and ends of your hair to nourish and detangle. Use a wide-tooth comb to minimize breakage while wet.

5. Heat Styling and Protection:

Minimize heat exposure from styling tools and protect your hair by:

i.   Using heat protectant products before styling. Always request for lower heat settings whenever you are using styling tools.

ii.   Embracing heatless styling methods like braiding or air-drying whenever possible.

6. Scalp Health:

i.   **Scalp Massages:** Incorporate scalp massages to stimulate blood flow and promote hair growth.

ii.   **Healthy Oils:** Use natural oils like coconut, argan, or jojoba to nourish the scalp and hair.

7. Protecting Hair:

i. **Treat Hair Gently:** Avoid vigorous towel-drying and rough handling of wet hair to prevent breakage.

ii. **Protective Styles:** Use gentle hair ties and embrace protective hairstyles to minimize stress on hair strands.

7. Stress Management:

Practice stress-reducing techniques like meditation, yoga, or hobbies to prevent stress-related hair issues.

8. Regular Trims:

Trim hair very few months to remove split ends and maintain hair health.

9. Environmental Protection:

Shield your hair from harsh weather conditions, sun exposure, and pollutants by wearing hats or using protective hair products.

10. Professional Care:

Seek professional advice from hair specialists or dermatologists for personalized care if facing persistent hair concerns.

By incorporating these healthy habits into your daily routine, you create a nurturing environment for your hair, fostering strength, shine, and overall hair health.

Choosing Natural Hair Care Products

Opting for natural hair care products can benefit your hair health while reducing exposure to potentially harsh chemicals. Understanding how to identify and select these products can contribute to maintaining healthier, more vibrant hair.

1. Understanding Ingredient Labels:

i. **Avoid Harsh Chemicals:** Look for products free from sulfates, parabens, phthalates, and silicones, as these can strip hair of natural oils and cause dryness.

ii.   **Botanical Ingredients:** Seek products containing natural botanical extracts like aloe vera, coconut oil, shea butter, argan oil, or essential oils.

2. Product Certifications:

Look for certifications such as USDA Organic, Ecocert, or COSMOS to ensure the product meets specific organic or natural standards.

3. Research and Reviews:

i. **Read Labels:** Carefully read product labels and research unfamiliar ingredients to understand their benefits or potential side effects.

ii. **Customer Reviews:** Consider customer reviews and feedback to gauge the effectiveness and suitability of the product for various hair types.

4. Hair Type Consideration:

HAIR GROWTH ELIXIR: 100% Natural Hair Growth Solution!

Select products tailored to your hair type, whether it's dry, oily, curly, straight, or color-treated, to address specific needs.

5. Trial and Patch Testing:

Conduct patch tests before using new products to check for any allergic reactions or adverse effects, especially if you have sensitive skin or scalp.

6. DIY and Homemade Remedies:

Consider creating your own hair care products using natural ingredients like avocado, honey, aloe vera, or apple cider vinegar. Homemade remedies offer customization and control over the ingredients used.

7. Transparency and Ethics:

HAIR GROWTH ELIXIR: 100% Natural Hair Growth Solution! Support brands that prioritize transparency regarding their sourcing, production methods, and commitment to sustainability and ethical practices.

8. Hair Styling Products:

For styling products like gels, mousses, or hairsprays, opt for natural alternatives without alcohol or synthetic fragrances that can be harsh on the hair and scalp.

9. Patience and Consistency:

Allow time for natural products to show their effects. Hair may require an adjustment period when transitioning from conventional to natural products.

11.Professional Advice:

Consult with a hair care professional for recommendations on natural products tailored to your specific hair concerns or conditions.

By being discerning about the ingredients, certifications, and suitability for your hair type, you can make informed choices when selecting natural hair care products. Over time, these products can contribute to healthier, more nourished, and vibrant hair.

Maintaining Long-Term Hair Health

Long-term hair health requires consistent care, healthy practices, and mindful routines that nourish and protect the hair and scalp. Adopting these habits contributes to resilient, vibrant hair in the long run.

1. Consistent and Gentle Care:

i. **Regular Washing:** Use a gentle, sulfate-free shampoo suitable for your hair type and avoid overwashing to preserve natural oils.

ii. **Proper Conditioning:** Apply conditioner to hydrate and detangle hair, focusing on the lengths and ends, and use a wide-tooth comb to minimize breakage.

2. Scalp Nourishment:

i. **Scalp Massages:** Incorporate scalp massages to stimulate blood flow, promoting a healthy environment for hair growth.

ii. **Scalp Treatments:** Use natural oils or serums to nourish the scalp and maintain its health.

3. Healthy Lifestyle Habits:

i. **Balanced Diet:** Consume a diet rich in proteins, vitamins (especially A, C, and E), minerals (like iron and zinc), and omega-3 fatty acids for overall hair health.

ii. **Hydration:** Stay well-hydrated by drinking enough water daily to keep the scalp and hair hydrated.

4. Protective Measures:

i. **Limit Heat Styling:** Minimize the use of heat styling tools and opt for air-drying or heatless styling methods whenever possible.

ii. **Protective Hairstyles:** Embrace hairstyles that minimize tension and stress on the hair, reducing breakage and damage.

5. Routine Trims and Maintenance:

i. **Regular Trims:** Schedule periodic trims to remove split ends and maintain healthy-looking hair.

ii. **Professional Consultation:** Seek advice from hair specialists or dermatologists to address any persistent issues or changes in hair health.

6. Stress Management:

i. **Stress Reduction Techniques:** Practice stress-relieving activities like meditation, yoga, or hobbies to mitigate stress-induced hair issues.

ii. **Adequate Sleep:** Prioritize quality sleep to support the body's natural repair processes, including those involved in hair health.

7. Choosing Natural Products:

Opt for natural and gentle hair care products free from harsh chemicals, prioritizing ingredients that nourish and protect the hair.

8. Weather and Environmental Protection:

i. **Protect from Sun and Pollution:** Use hats or scarves to shield hair from harsh sun exposure and pollutants.

ii. Moisture and Hydration: Adjust hair care routines seasonally to counteract the effects of weather changes, ensuring adequate hydration and protection.

9. Consistency and Patience:

Maintain a consistent hair care routine and be patient with natural remedies or treatments, as results may take time to show.

By incorporating these practices into your lifestyle and being mindful of the needs of your hair and scalp, you can maintain long-term hair health, promoting resilience, strength, and vibrancy.

ABOUT THE BOOK

HAIR GROWTH ELIXIR: 100% Natural Hair Growth Solution! is a comprehensive guide dedicated to helping you nurture healthy hair growth using natural and holistic approaches. This book offers a wealth of knowledge, encompassing various aspects of hair care, scalp health, and lifestyle practices tailored to foster robust and vibrant hair.

In this guide, the author will journey you through hair growth cycles, the factors influencing hair health, the importance of personalized hair care, from the fundamental principles of scalp care to identifying herbal remedies, essential oils, and DIY treatments, hair nutrition, stress management, herbal treatments, and scalp care techniques, It emphasizes the significance of a balanced lifestyle, gentle hair care practices, and the selection of natural products to promote long-term hair health and vitality.

www.ingramcontent.com/pod-product-compliance
Lightning Source LLC
Chambersburg PA
CBHW060955260726
48661CB00005B/1890